A LIFE ON

CIGARETTES

Smoking, Smoking Hazards,

And Consequences

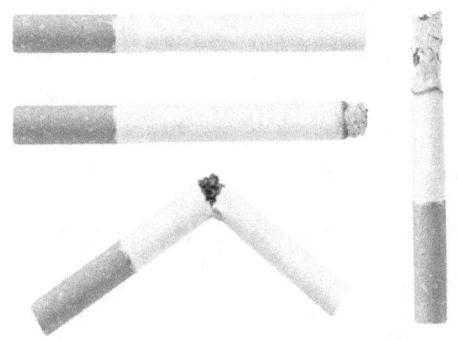

By

Paolo Jose de Luna

Table of Contents

INTRODUCTION

Smoking: Then and Now

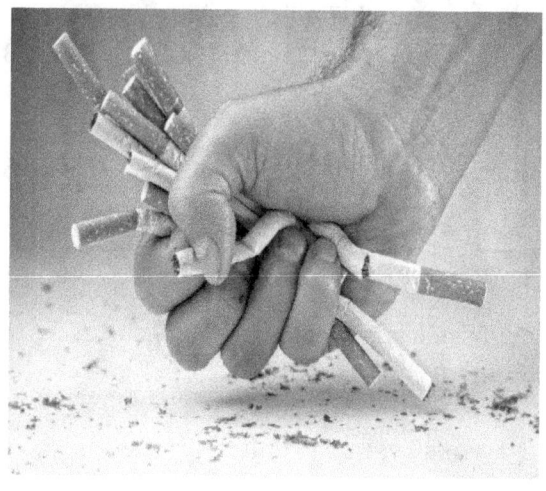

The first recorded practice of smoking dates back as far as 5000 BC up to 3000 BC. It was when cultivation of crops in South America started and the consumption of those crops later led to the practice of burning the plant substance, whether it was by accident or with intent, it worked its way to be included in the shamanistic rituals of our prehistoric ancestors and it was that sort of practice that gave way for raising tobacco as a type of crop. Later on, various civilizations like the Indians, the Babylonians, and the Chinese had this practice of burning incense during their religious rituals, which was then later adapted by the Christians.It has been speculated that burning incense influenced the practice of smoking in the Americas from their origins of the shamanistic rituals, but was later adapted into a practice for pleasure, leisure, or as a social tool. The practice of smoking tobacco and various hallucinogenic drugs were done to achieve a state of trance or "high" as they call it to contact the spirit world.

It was in 1612 when John Rolfe turned tobacco into a real cash crop. With the demand for tobacco rising through the roof, past Rolfe's expectations, tobacco was then referred to as the "browned gold" since it revived the Virginia joint stock company that failed because of its fruitless gold expeditions. And in order to meet that demand, tobacco was then grown in continuous succession, rapidly depleting the soil from its nutrients and crashing the overall quality of the soil.

In 2006, the number of those who are still smoking in the US fell from 42% to a mere 20.8% and most of those who quit smoking were mostly professional and wealthy men. However, that still isn't good enough when it comes to the practice of smoking. That's because even though the number of those who are smoking decreased, the average number of cigarettes consumed by each smoker each day drastically increased from 20 up to 30 cigarette sticks per day. That would mean those who didn't quit smoking ended up smoking more cigarettes each day. Even today, Russia is the leading consumer when it comes to cigarettes, closely followed by countries like Laos, Ukraine, Indonesia, Jordan, Greece, and China.

Are you planning on quitting smoking? Do you have a family member or a loved one that you want to stop smoking? Well, this is the book for you! In this book, we'll be learning more about smoking, the practice, the various contents of a cigarette stick, and the health hazards involved in partaking in the practice of smoking. Hold on to your seat as you'll be getting the most straightforward facts, truths, and details on smoking that will shake your beliefs.

Chapter 1 - The Practice of Smoking

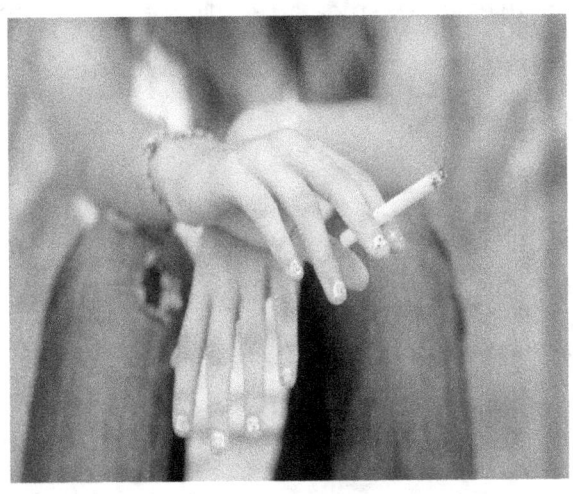

Smoking has been around literally for centuries. Dating as far back as 5000 BC, the practice of smoking was primarily discovered for religious and shamanistic practices to get into a state of trance and establish contact with the spirit world. However, as years went by, smoking was then used for leisure, pleasure, and as a social activity. It was at this turning point in history when the term "moderation" for smoking died out. Once it was used for leisure and pleasure, there was no stopping various people in whiffing out their cigarettes.

Tobacco and cigarette smoking are widely related because the concept behind them is exactly the same, though the apparatus used may be different.

Tobacco smoking involves the use of a pipe that is often handmade or crafted from various types of materials like wood, steel, or plastic. With one end of the pipe meant for the mouth while the other end meant for stuffing the dried tobacco leaves, the leaves are burnt to produce smoke which is then consumed by the smoker.

But compared to tobacco smoking, cigarettes are a whole lot easier.

With cigarette smoking, you already get a ready-made tobacco complete with pipe and tobacco leaves. Cigarette sticks often come in white and then about a fourth of the stick has a different shade of color depending on the manufacturer brand or even the flavor of the cigarette which can range from green, red, brown, yellow, or gold. To smoke a cigarette stick, all you have to do is to put one end of the cigarette onto your mouth, light the other end of the stick with a lighter or a match, and then you're good to go in consuming your smoke.

It's because smoking has become so easy that a lot of people are still using it and a lot more people end up smoking ore cigarette sticks than they used to years ago. What's alarming about smoking is that not only does the average number of sticks a usual smoker consumes each day, the age that when people start to smoke is growing younger and younger with each passing moment. Back then, smoking was just something done by adults. Years later, smoking was then passed on to college kids. Eventually, smoking has reached as far as high school kids that it isn't something new to see a high school kid smoking a stick of cigarette. However, what's really alarming now is to see kids as young as 10 or even younger to smoke a stick of cigarette without a care in the world.

That brings us to another critical question – why do kids end up smoking? Why do kids choose to smoke? Do they have a choice or is it out of mere impulse? Do they get hooked to the addictiveness that cigarettes have to offer or do they get pressured by their social peers?

A lot of reasons come into play when it comes to why people end up smoking. Most often, people engage in smoking after being influenced by their parents or their friends, but mostly by friends. The earlier a person starts smoking, the higher chance that they'll be continuing smoking even into adulthood or maybe even through their retirement years.

However, one thing is for certain – the degradation of smoking from being a ritualistic practice for religious and shamanistic purposes into an activity for leisure and pleasure has made it accessible for the younger generation to do it without regard and care about the consequences that it brings. "Irresponsible smoking" as many would dub it, puts great risk to our health, both for the smokers and those around the smokers, as well as the environment.

With every year that passes, the practice of smoking is evolving with the times, whether it is for better or worse. Some of the biggest cigarette manufacturers have extended their reach to smokers by providing the newest flavors of cigarettes while some manufacturers have opted to see the light and provide something as an alternative that's healthier and cheaper compared to the traditional way of smoking.

But the decision still lies within you.

Will you risk the health of your family, friends, and loved ones, as well as your own, or will you change for the better and quit smoking once and for all? It isn't an easy thing to do and it will definitely take a lot of time to getting used to and battling out of addiction.

But one thing's for certain – it is possible.

Chapter 2 - Why Do People Smoke?

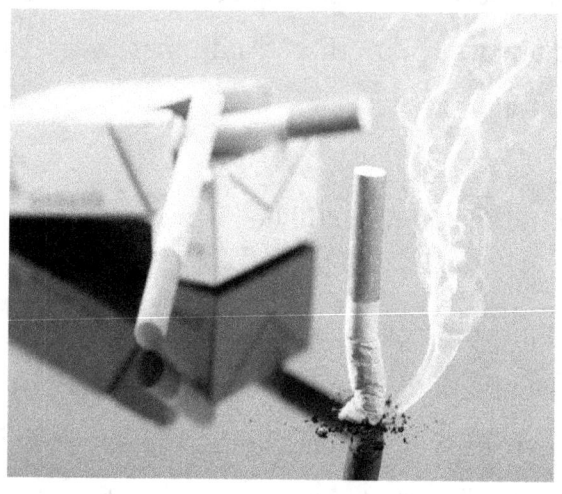

There are various reasons as to why people start smoking. Most often, people start smoking during their teenage years. By the time they reach adulthood, they're already addicted to cigarettes and by that point in time, it's already hard to quit smoking because of the substance, *nicotine*. But what compels most people to start smoking in the first place? Here are the following reasons:

Peer Pressure

Let's first begin where the roots of smoking are – the teenage years. If you ask most smokers the first time when they started smoking, they're probably going to answer during their teenage years. While just one of the many reasons as to why people start to smoke, peer pressure certainly plays a big role. During these years of adjustment and self-searching, adolescents are prone to the influence of their friends, rather than their parents. Trying cigarettes through the experimentation period of many teenagers proves to be a strong foundation of addiction.

Eventually, the smoker shares his or her experience to friends to expand the boundaries. Those who still haven't tried smoking are afraid to be branded by their smoker friends as afraid to take risks or extend their boundaries. Afraid of being left out, those who didn't smoke are convinced to smoke and later on, getting addicted to cigarettes.

Stress Relief

Probably the biggest reason as to why people start smoking, stress relief is a mainstay factor that seems to hard to eradicate. It was during the World War when soldier smoked cigars and tobacco to battled wartime stress and the psychological turmoil that they experienced during those times. However, many people who experience low-level stress like at work may start to smoke to provide relief for stress and to ease their nerves.

However, the problem now is that most people have a hard time quitting cigarettes even after the stress has passed. It becomes some sort of psychological and chemical crutch that one becomes dependent upon and at times, one can't even function without smoking a cigarette first. That's because once a stressful situation hits them, they reach out for a cigarette out of instinct. And eventually, the thing that relieved their stress becomes the very source of their stress.

Family Influence

Studies have shown that children who have smoker parents have a higher tendency to smoke cigarettes by the time they reach their adolescent period. Parental influence plays a big role in the practice of smoking in children and in the worse case scenario, some children even begin smoking during their school age years provided that their parents don't give them adequate guidance and supervision.

However, it's not just for parents who smoke that children gain the tendency to smoke. Parents who also accept smoking as an agreeable behavior and allow their children to watch movies or TV shows that depict heavy use of cigarettes and alcohol increase the likelihood for their children to take up smoking. This just goes to show that the role of the family is important in preventing children to take up smoking.

Controlling Weight

Aside from stress relief, one of the reasons why people smoke cigarettes is to control their weight. That's because smoking suppresses the appetite of a person, preventing the smoker to eat more. Cigarettes also lessen a person's sense of taste and smell, so stimulation from aromatic food might not have a significant effect to a smoker's appetite. That's also the reason why a lot of smokers tend to gain weight when they start to quit smoking because their appetite is stimulated.

However, when you think about it, there are a lot of ways that you can suppress your appetite and control your weight. Good examples would be drinking a full glass of water before every meal, engaging in exercise, and choosing a healthy diet comprised mostly of fruits and vegetables. Through these various methods, you don't need to damage your body through smoking just for the sake of controlling your weight.

An Attempt to Look Mature

People have this inclination to try and look cool towards their peers. Especially true for adolescents, trying to look mature is one of the main reasons as to why people try out and experiment on smoking cigarettes. Being accepted by their peers and getting recognition for it is a big hit for adolescents. Being seen as "mature" by their peers and other people is something important to them in this period of self-searching and establishing their own identity.

However, this should not be the case. With proper parental guidance and education, trying to look mature by smoking cigarettes shouldn't be the solution. In fact, promoting self-independence by letting teenagers make their own decisions like deciding what college or university they want to go to, what movie they want to watch, what games they want to play, or what job that they want to have. A parent's role should be as someone who guides, rather than someone who controls. While you can give your opinions and insights, let your child be the one to decide and respect their decision. Provide choices for your child and allow them to make their own decisions.

Taking Risks

Some people gain self-gratification by breaking the rules. There are a lot of countries where adults put their eyebrows together because of all the signs that say "No Smoking" scattered all over cities and public establishments. Because of this prohibition, it's quite difficult to smoke in public places, including the streets because authorities may walk up to you and give you a good reprimand.

However, there's a thrill from breaking those set of rules. This is especially true for teenagers who are still undergoing a rebellious stage in an attempt to act cool and tough in front of their peers by breaking the rules set by their school, their parents, and their community. And it comes as no surprise that most teenagers push things to the limit and try smoking in secrecy and gain a sense of high just by breaking the rules as they feel a sense of adrenaline and excitement, knowing that what they're doing is against the norm.

There are certainly a lot of reasons as to why people start smoking. May it be from stress, may it be from a medical condition, may it be out of peer pressure, smoking can still be avoided through one thing and one thing only – choice. While there are some factors that come into play for some people when it comes to the practice of smoking, it's still your choice whether or not you're going to engage in this unhealthy practice.

Education and parental guidance are essential support systems that can prevent people from smoking in the first place, especially for teenagers. Because with aadequate knowledge and support, giving in to this addictive practice won't be easy as it is now.

Chapter 3 - The Contents of a Cigarette

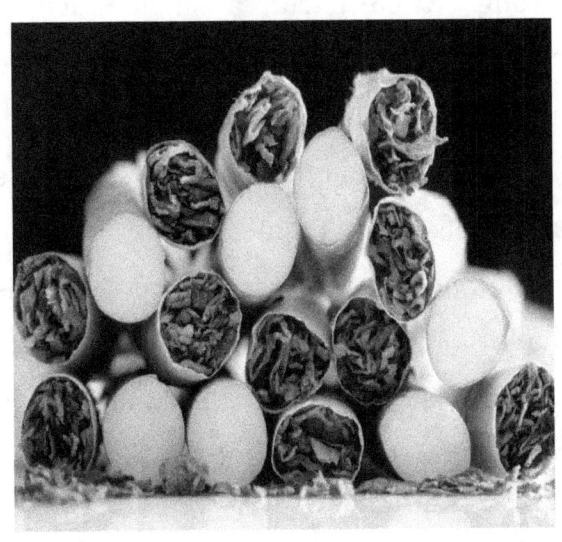

You may not be aware of it, but did you know that there are over 600 active ingredients in just one stick of cigarette? Yes, you've got that right. There are more than 600 ingredients in one stick of cigarette and all of them bring harm to the smoker, to those around the smoker, and the environment.

But it doesn't stop there. You're dead wrong. When burnt, a single stick of cigarette can produce as much as 7,000 chemicals that are harmful to your health and those around the smoker. These chemicals aren't meant for human consumption and constant reminder is made by cigarette manufacturing companies to smoke in moderation because of these chemicals. That's also the reason why you can see a lot of chemical residues in the lungs of a smoker, even sticking to the phlegm that is often hacked up by the average smoker.

Here are just some of the chemicals that can be found in single stick of cigarette and what they are that you need to watch out for in the first place.

Arsenic

Let's start off with the big bomb here. One of the main ingredients that can be found in cigarette is arsenic which is known to be used in rat poison and other pesticides. You've got that right – RAT POISON. If you're smoking cigarette, you're just whiffing a good dose of rat poison. No wonder that your lungs take a beating when you smoke. So if that isn't enough to convince you to stop smoking, then you've got to set your priorities straight.

Benzene

A chemical found in rubber cement, benzene is the binding chemical that lets rubber cement stick together. When inhaled, such as in the form of cigarette smoke, benzene leaves gooey residue in the lungs, specifically in the alveoli, destroying the lung tissue overtime and reduces the total volume of air that you can inhale with your lungs.

Butane

Another dangerous chemical in cigarette, butane can be found in lighter fluid. It's flammable which helps light up the cigarette with just a small light. However, the biggest issue that butane can cause is that it's dangerously cancerous when consumed by the body. In fact, butane can "melt" the cells in your lungs through continuous smoking and consumption of butane.

Lead

Used in dry cell batteries, lead is known for being poisonous. A lot of products that contain lead are often pulled out from the market because of the danger of lead poisoning. However, cigarette is known to carry lead and can even risk children to develop psychological problems and pregnant women to have a higher rate of abortion.

Naphthalene

Ever wondered why the smell of cigarette smoke can sometimes be bitter or a bit minty? Well, that's because it contains naphthalene, the same thing that is also contained in moth balls. The unique chemical called naphthalene is used as a primary ingredient in moth balls to kill moths, cockroaches, and other pests from clothes. If you're smoking, you're just consuming a dose of moth ball with each stick of cigarette.

Formaldehyde

Another cancerous substance, formaldehyde is used as a chemical to preserve body parts, corpses, and animals. When inhaled, it can be very damaging to the lungs, the throat, and the nose. As a pure chemical that is often called "formalin", this chemical can cause painful stimuli when inhaled directly and its damaging effects are not mitigated with its inclusion in cigarettes.

Cadmium

Being an active component in battery acid, cadmium can be very damaging to the lungs. When included in cigarettes, cadmium can also damage the alveoli and the nerves along the airway.

Carbon Monoxide

Carbon monoxide is known as a gaseous poison that has left an onslaught of victims because of how deadly it is. It is often release in a car's exhaust fumes and the deadly effects that carbon monoxide can bring result in tightening of the airways and suffocation.

Acetone

Found in nail polish remover, acetone can also be damaging to the airway and the lungs. When inhaled, it can cause pain and lung damage, especially through prolonged consumption.

Ammonia

Used in most common household cleaners, ammonia is a deadly chemical when consumed inappropriately.

Hexamine

Another flammable liquid in cigarettes, hexamine is used in barbecue lighter fluid and provides the flammable properties of a cigarette. When consumed through cigarette, hexamine damages the lungs and the airway.

Tar

A chemical that's often used to pave roads, tar leaves black residual content on the lungs which results in irreversible lung damage that can be seen through diagnostic procedures and is an obvious sight when doing the autopsy of a chain smoker's lungs.

Toluene

Toluene is a chemical that's often found in manufacture paint and paint is something that can easily damage the airways when smelled for a long time. Imagine that when consuming cigarettes and it's like you're sniffing paint on a continuous basis and you're just asking your lungs to get damaged overtime.

Nicotine

Last but definitely not the least; this is the thing that keeps you getting hooked on smoking cigarettes even if you know that it's bad for your health. Nicotine is the addictive substance that forces you to keep coming back to cigs and the very reason why it's difficult to quit smoking cigarettes in the first place. Did you also know that nicotine is also used in pesticides and insecticides? So yeah, you're practically killing yourself with a pesticide when you smoke a cigarette.

There are certainly more chemicals that you can find in cigarettes. Those mentioned here are just the tip of the iceberg, but not one of them are considered good for your body. Most of these chemicals, if not all, are considered harmful to the body. In fact, most of these chemicals are cancerous and shouldn't be consumed in the first place!

Sure, you may control your appetite and you may control your weight when you smoke, but that's nothing compared to the consequences that you'll be getting in terms of your health and the health of other people when you smoke a cigarette. A cigarette stick is just a concoction of pure danger, putting your health and the health of everyone you love at risk. If you don't want to take that risk, then think about everything that you know about smoking so far and start weighing the consequences.

Chapter 4 - The Health Effects of Smoking

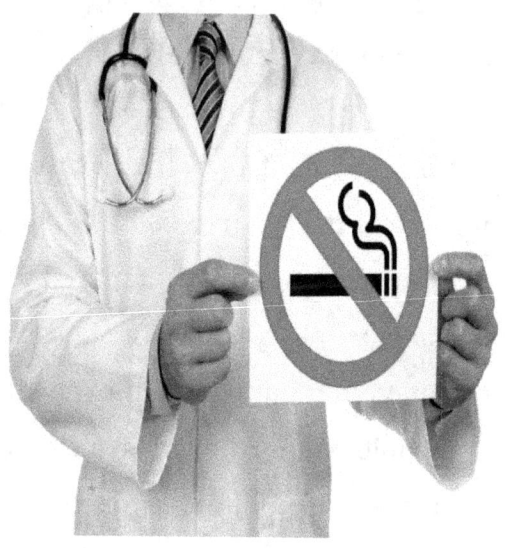

After know the basics of smoking and the contents of a single cigarette stick, it's time to know the implications when it comes to your health with each stick that you consume. You've probably heard countless of doctors and nurses strongly advise you or other people to stop smoking – not just reduce, not just lessen, but to STOP. That's because smoking won't do you any good in terms of your health. It may be used to ease your nerves, but you'll end up regretting it once it comes to your health. Smoking is one of the biggest factors when it comes to the development of various diseases and health conditions. Some don't even come from the smoker, as there are also a lot of health conditions that come from inhaling second-hand smoke, so be aware, be concerned, and be knowledgeable on the effects of smoking on our health.

Cancer

Smoking is one of the biggest factors when it comes to cancer. Lung cancer is the most likely form of cancer to develop in smokers, but other forms of cancer can also develop particularly laryngeal cancer, renal cancer, cancer of the head and neck, bladder cancer, liver cancer, esophageal cancer, pancreatic cancer, and gastric cancer. Studies have shown that cigarette smoking, even second-hand smoke, increases the likelihood for cancer to develop in both men and women, specifically cervical cancer for females. There are also some studies that prove that smoking can also contribute to the development of squamous cell carcinoma, colorectal cancer, intestinal cancer, breast cancer, and leukemia.

Pulmonary Problems

Because of the usual way cigarettes are consumed, it's expected that pulmonary problems will develop overtime. Some of the most common pulmonary health conditions that can be seen in a lot of smokers include bronchitis, asthma, emphysema, pneumonia, lung cancer, tuberculosis, and chronic obstructive pulmonary disease (COPD), which are all equally as dangerous and equally as expensive when it comes to their treatment. If you don't want to develop these sorts of health problems, then it's time to stop smoking once and for all.

Cardiovascular Problems

Aside from pulmonary problems, smokers are also at risk for developing health conditions involving the heart and the cardiovascular system. These would include problems like atherosclerosis, high blood pressure, myocardial infarction, coronary artery disease, and stroke. Studies have found out that there has been a high incidence of heart attacks among smokers because the chemicals in cigarettes cause the blood vessels to constrict, resulting in an increased blood pressure, sometimes even at dangerously high levels, and even causing the heart to lose its supply of oxygen.

Nervous System Problems

Smokers are generally at a greater risk when it comes to developing stroke, Alzheimer's, dementia, encephalitis, brain tumors, and other neurologic problems. The chemicals contained in cigarettes give way to damage the brain cells and when these chemicals cross the blood-brain barrier, it can cause irreversible damage to the brain. Aside from the brain, the spinal cord is also affected as the contents of cigarettes can also damage the spinal cord and destroy the fine lining of the nerves.

Kidney Problems

Research has also shown that smokers are significantly at risk in developing renal problems including cancer in the kidneys and the bladder. Aside from cancer, smokers are also more prone to develop urinary tract infections, kidney stones, renal trauma, and more.

Infections and Immune System Problems

Smokers are generally at a greater risk to develop infections. That's because the chemicals in cigarette suppress or decrease the overall defense of the immune system, making way for various infections to develop. Infections like influenza, pneumonia, tuberculosis, urinary tract infection, encephalitis, and other types of infection can develop in those who smoke, particularly chain smokers. Keep in mind that infections are hard and very expensive to treat because of the antibiotic that you need to take, so if you don't want to suffer from these various forms and infection and if you don't want your wallet to empty out, then steer clear when it comes to smoking.

Impotence and Infertility

Smoking is one of the biggest factors when it comes to the development of impotence. In fact, about 85% of smokers are prone to become impotent after a few years and smoking is also a key factor in the incidence of erectile dysfunction. That's because cigarette smoke promotes the narrowing of the arteries which lessens the blood supply to the reproductive organs and even affects the supply of oxygen to these organs. A low sperm count among males is also found in those who keep smoking. Female infertility is also found among female smokers because the chemicals in cigarettes alter the production of the female hormone, estrogen which has a key role in ovulation. Smoking is also a big determinant for various forms of abortion and fetal abnormalities, particularly if the pregnant woman is a smoker or is in the frequent vicinity of a smoker. Cigarettes are known as teratogenic agents that promote abortion and can leave permanent disabilities in the fetus by the time they are born.

Psychological Effects

Research has found out that various psychological problems are prone to develop in those who smoke. Depression and aggression are found to be common among smokers because of the stress that they experience, especially when they have been used to the stress-relieving effects of cigarettes that their bodies forget this type of benefit that smoking brings. It has also been found out that smoking gives way to cognitive dysfunction, further increasing the risk in the development of Alzheimer's disease. Withdrawal symptoms can also be observed in those who don't get their daily fix of cigarette which gets worse the longer a person is fixated on smoking, similar to excessive alcohol consumption. The development of schizophrenia is also correlated to cigarette smoking because of the chemicals that can damage the brain cells and alter the production of neurotransmitters in the brain.

The harm and consequences of smoking certainly opens up the true nature of this long-standing practice. While it may bring stress relief and relaxation, these seemingly positive effects of smoking are only temporary. That eradicates the benefits because smoking leaves lifelong harm and consequences to the body that may take from months to years to show up. And by the times the signs and symptoms of these health conditions shows up, it might be already too late for you or one of your loved ones who were exposed to cigarette smoke. So if you don't want to develop any of these health problems for yourself or anyone you care about, then it's time to quit smoking once and for all.

CONCLUSION

Smoking has been around for centuries. Coming from our ancestors of the past, it's no surprise that this sort of practice still exists in our modern time. Back then, smoking was just meant to be used for religious purposes and shamanistic rituals to contact the dead, establish a connection with the spirit world, or maybe even both. However, through the hundreds of years that passed by, the practice of smoking shifted towards an activity of leisure and social gathering. And it was because of this change that smoking has become an unhealthy habit that we know all too well today.

There are a lot of factors that come into play as to why people start smoking. Most usually, people start smoking during their teenage years when the social influence from peers is at its strongest. Smoking becomes a form of self-reliance in an attempt to look mature among teenagers, but most adolescents don't understand the risks and consequences of smoking at their age.

While some smokers may claim that smoking a cigar or two can help relieve the stress and ease their nerves, the harm clearly outweighs all the benefits. There are various health conditions that can develop overtime, particularly for those who start smoking at an earlier age.

When it comes to smoking, one word manages to come into mind – cancer. Smokers are more prone to develop various forms of cancer because of all the chemicals that they consume. That's because cigarettes and tobacco by themselves are considered as cancerous agents. The chemicals contained in cigarettes are considered as cancerous and some are not even meant to be consumed by the human body. Once consumed, these chemicals do significant harm to the body, leaving evident traces of damage overtime.

But the health risk is not just your own. Smoking also risks the health of everyone around you. Think of your mom, your dad, your siblings, your wife, or your children. Smoking hits them all and if you don't do anything about it, they may be first on the list to develop the various health problems that we've just discussed earlier. If you care about your family, if you care about your loved ones, you will know what you have to do and you will take a stand on what decision that you have to make.

So now, what do you want to do? Will you keep on smoking that stick of cigarette, knowing all too well of the health risks and knowing that it won't be just you suffering, or will you make the smart choice of putting down that stick and stop smoking once and for all? So what's it going to be? Weigh everything that you have and think about it. The decision lies within you and you alone.